Idiopathic Thrombocytopenic Purpura (ITP)
Fast Focus Study Guide

JT Thomas, MD

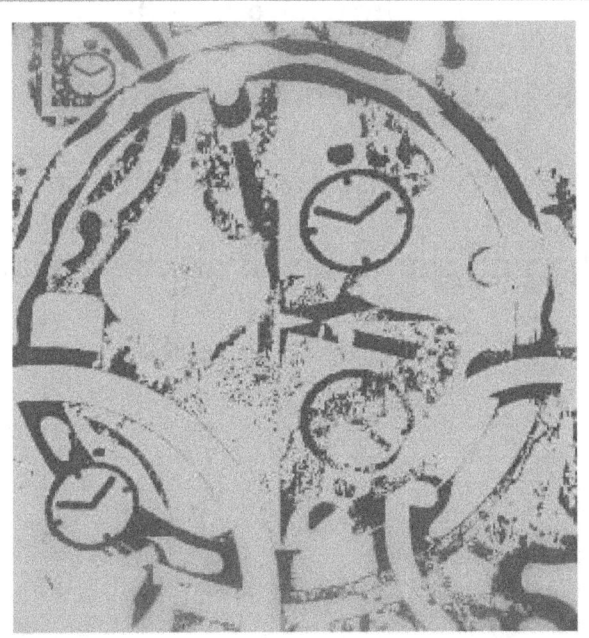

Acknowledgements

I dedicate this book to my beautiful wife and children, who I love more than all the water in all the oceans and all the seas.

CONTENTS

- This book is written to help the reader further understand Idiopathic Thrombocytopenic Purpura (ITP).

- This book is written in a simple and easy to read format designed for medical students, residents and physicians who are preparing for boards.

- This book simplifies a complicated medical issue so you will remember the important details.

- You will not get caught up in the minutia. Just the facts are found in this book.

- This Fast Focus Study Guide will provide you with a practical review of the key information you need to know.

- Buy this book now if you want this quick and concise information

Immune thrombocytopenia (ITP) is a condition that is characterized by antibody-mediated destruction of platelets associated with impaired megakaryocyte platelet production.

Incidence

The incidence of ITP in adults is 1.6-6.6 per
100,000

Incidence

There are peaks in the incidence in patients younger than age 40 y/o with a female predominance and a second peak incidence in patients older than 60 y/o with no gender predominance.

Treatment

Patients with ITP should stop all NSAIDS and ASA to improve platelet function.

Pathophysiology

In patients the lifespan of the platelet is significantly less than normal platelet lifespan is 10 days.

Idiopathic Thrombocytopenic Purpura (ITP) is an illness that occurs in an otherwise healthy person.

Signs and Symptoms

The typical patient with ITP does not have signs or symptoms of infection, weight loss lymphadenopathy, or chronic illness.

Pathophysiology of ITP

It is thought that people with ITP have for some reason made an antibody that cross reacts with the platelets when the immune system loses tolerance to self-antigens located on the surface of the platelets and megakaryocytes.

The antiplatelet antibodies are produced by B cells and are known to target primary platelet glycoproteins such as GP IIb/ IIIa.

The antiplatelet antibodies have effects on circulating platelets and also effect platelet glycoproteins on the surface of megakaryocytes causing destruction and decreased platelet production.

The antibody coated platelets bound by are removed by Fc receptors on splenic macrophages.

Pathophysiology of ITP

Thrombocytopenia is mediated by immune directed destruction of immunoglobulin-coated platelets in patients with ITP. This is mediated by macrophage IgG Fc (Fc gamma RI, Fc gamma RII, and Fc gamma RIII) and complement receptors (CR1, CR3).

Pathophysiology of ITP

The spleen contributes to autoantibody production and phagocytosis of antibody coated platelets in patients with ITP.

Pathophysiology of ITP

About 75% of autoantibodies present in patients with chronic ITP are directed against platelet GPIIb/IIIa or GPIb/IX GP complexes, with the remaining patients likely having antibodies against other membrane epitopes, including GPV, GPIa/IIa, or GPIV.

Pathophysiology of ITP

Splenic macrophages are responsible for removing platelets in patients with ITP therefore splenectomy often results in quick restoration of normal platelet counts in most patients with ITP.

Most patients with ITP will have minimal bleeding as long as the platelet count if > 30,000/L.

Viruses Associated with ITP

It is not unusual for patients with a new diagnosis of ITP to describe a recent history of an antecedent viral gastroenteritis or upper respiratory infection.

Signs and Symptoms

You can often determine the severity of ITP with a simple skin and mucous membrane examination.

Signs and Symptoms

If a patient with presumed ITP presents a
severe thrombocytopenia associated with
diffuse petechia, widespread ecchymosis,
gingival bleeding, or hemorrhagic bullae, the
patient is at risk for a serious bleeding
complication.

Signs and Symptoms

The typical patient with ITP does not have signs or symptoms of infection, weight loss lymphadenopathy, or chronic illness.

Symptoms

The most common symptoms of ITP can include hemorrhage, petechiae, purpura, epistaxis, gingival bleeding, menorrhagia, and easy bruising.

Symptoms

Hematuria, GI bleeding, retinal hemorrhage, and even intracranial bleeding can be seen rarely in patients with severe ITP.

Signs and Symptoms

The finding of splenomegaly is inconsistent with ITP may indicate chronic liver disease or lymphoma.

Signs and Symptoms

If examination of a patient with suspected ITP reveals asymmetrical neurologic findings, then intracranial hemorrhage could be present.

Differential Diagnosis

The differential diagnosis of isolated thrombocytopenia includes pseudothrombocytopenia, TTP, DIC, SLE, antiphospholipid antibody syndrome, HIV, HCV, EBV, CLL, lymphoma, large granular lymphocytic leukemia, myelodysplasia, splenomegaly, pregnancy associated thrombocytopenia, and transfusion reaction. Drugs that can cause these findings include heparin, quinidine, sulfa, and gold, alcohol. Less common causes can include Wiskott-Aldrich, Bernard-Soulier, Fanconi's anemia, and pure megakaryocyte aplasia.

Viruses Associated with ITP

There are several viruses that are associated with ITP including EBV, CMV, Varicella, Rubella, as well as Hepatitis A, B, and C.

Risk Factors

Thrombocytopenia in the setting of Hepatitis C is multifactorial and likely related to bone marrow suppression, auto antibodies, hypersplenism, antiviral therapy and decreased thrombopoietin levels.

In patients with splenomegaly related to cirrhosis and portal hypertension there is pooling of platelets within an enlarged spleen

Thrombocytopenia can occur in the setting of cirrhosis without splenomegaly due to decreased production of thrombopoietin from the liver and decreased production of platelets within the bone marrow.

Alcohol

Thrombocytopenia can occur in patients with alcoholism even in those without associated liver disease due to generalized suppression by alcohol on blood cell production within the bone marrow.

Hepatitis C and Thrombocytopenia

Thrombocytopenia in patients with hepatitis C can be related to bone marrow inhibition related to direct infection of megakaryocytes or decreased thrombopoietin production by the liver.

Medications Associated with ITP

There are over 1400 drugs listed in the United States FDA Adverse Event Reporting System database associated with thrombocytopenia.

Medications Associated with ITP

Some of the most common drugs associated with thrombocytopenia are listed on the next page.

Risk Factors

An autoimmune disorder can be suspected in patients who have a history of illness characterized by chronic and recurring symptoms. These symptoms could include painful, tender, or swollen joints.

Risk Factors

In the United States H pylori infections do
not appear to be associated with increased risk
of ITP.

Assays for platelet-associated immunoglobulin (Antiplatelet antibody) by ELISA or flow cytometry may be positive, but these assays are not part of the recommended workup due to unreliable results and poor sensitivity.

Bone Marrow

Bone marrow is not always done, but sometimes it is needed to evaluate patients who do not clearly fit the diagnosis of ITP.

Testing

Since HIV and Hepatitis C can be associated with ITP, serologic testing for HIV and hepatitis C should be considered.

Workup

The most important tests in patients with suspected ITP include the CBC with differential and peripheral smear, HIV, and bone marrow biopsy testing patients older than 60.

Viruses Associated with ITP

There are several viruses that are associated with ITP including EBV, CMV, Varicella, Rubella, as well as Hepatitis A, B, and C.

Testing

The peripheral blood smear examination is
done to evaluate red cell morphology.
Microscopic examination is done to find
schistocytes or reticulocytes that might be seen
in a microangiopathic hemolytic anemia.
White cells are visualized to ensure that there
is no evidence of leukemia or myelodysplasia.

Testing

Coagulation assays should be within normal limits in the setting of ITP.

Blood Tests

The LDH is often elevated in patients with lymphoma or leukemia and typically is not elevated in patients with ITP.

Blood Tests

Autoimmune disorders can be associated with ITP, therefore an ANA and rheumatoid factor studies can be done.

Blood Tests

Liver function tests and a pregnancy test can be sent since thrombocytopenia can be associated with chronic liver disease and pregnancy.

Blood Tests

The D-dimer and FDP assay help to rule out DIC as the cause of ITP.

Blood Tests

The peripheral smear will also evaluate for pseudothrombocytopenia that is characterized by platelet clumping.

Bone Marrow

A bone marrow aspirate and biopsy is characterized by normal or increased number of megakaryocytes in the absence of other significant abnormalities.

Bone Marrow

If the diagnosis of ITP is not clear, a bone marrow aspirate and biopsy is done to exclude myelodysplastic syndrome or leukemia.

Bone Marrow

The bone marrow aspiration and biopsy should be done to diagnose bone marrow hypoplasia or fibrosis prior to splenectomy.

Bone Marrow

On bone marrow examination, the cell concentration and morphology is normal. The megakaryocyte numbers are normal or increased. The megakaryocytes may be normal but sometimes are large and immature. There should be no dysplastic changes.

Corticosteroids

Treatment with prednisone, methylprednisolone, or high-dose dexamethasone is the initial treatment of choice for acute ITP.

IVIG and Rho Immunoglobulin

IV immunoglobulin (IVIG) or IV Rho immunoglobulin (Rh(D)-positive) are the standard second line treatments for patients with ITP who have not undergone splenectomy.

Treatment

There is a black-box warning for Rho immunoglobulin because of risk for intravascular hemolysis, acute renal failure, and DIC given to patients for ITP.

Treatment

In addition to IVIG and WinRho are standard first line treatments. Other options include splenectomy, rituximab, and the thrombopoietin-receptor agonists (TPO-RAs).

TPO Mimetics

Thrombopoietin (TPO) is a protein produced in the liver that controls how many platelets are made by megakaryocytes. The pharmaceutical companies can now produce TPO mimetics in the lab that can be used for treatment of ITP.

Treatment

Adults with a platelet count of $\geq$50,000 usually do not need treatment because they generally have minimal purpura and are at low risk of severe hemorrhage.

Transfusions

Platelet transfusions can be used in the setting of significant bleeding. The transfused platelets will have a shorter half-life than normally expected because of the underlying ITP.

Rituximab

Patients with a new diagnosis of ITP were randomized in a clinical trial to receive dexamethasone (40 mg/day × 4days) or dexamethasone with rituximab (375 mg/m2/week for 4 weeks). The trial found that 58% of the patients receiving rituximab and dexamethasone and in 37% of the group with dexamethasone alone had a platelet count > 50,000/L at 6 months.

Treatment

In another trial they used low-dose rituximab (100 mg/ dose × 4 doses) administered with dexamethasone. The 6-month sustained remission rate was 76.2%.

Splenectomy

Splenectomy can potentially cure ITP by removing the site of platelet destruction along with a source of antiplatelet antibody production.

Treatment

Splenectomy in patients with ITP produces a long term response rate approximately of 66%.

Treatment

Romiplostim and eltrombopag treats ITP by increasing the production of platelets through stimulating the thrombopoietin receptor.

Treatment

In a clinical trial, Romiplostim produced a platelet count $\geq$ 50,000/L during 6 or more of the 8 weeks of treatment in 38% of the splenectomized patients and 61% of the nonsplenectomized patients.

Treatment

Approximately 59%-81% of patients given the Eltrombopag had a platelet count of $\geq$ 50,000/L on day 43 compared with 11% to 16% of the patients given placebo.

Treatment

The EXTEND study demonstrated that eltrombopag produced a platelet count $\geq$ 50,000/L in > 50% of the patient visits.

Treatment

It is though that TPO-RAs can restore immune tolerance by improving T-regulatory function. This can result in sustained remission in a small percentage of patients after therapy is discontinued.

Treatment

Eltrombopag has a black box warning for hepatotoxicity. In the EXTEND study, 10% of patients developed drug-induced liver insufficiency. Approximately 66% of those patients had resolution of abnormalities after eltrombopag was stopped.

Treatment

The incidence of hemolytic reactions associated with Rho immunoglobulin is estimated at 1 in 1115 patients. These reactions occurred within 4 hours 94% of the time. The risk factors of acute hemolytic reactions include age > 65 years of age, renal dysfunction, current or recent infection including EBV.

Treatment

Potential side effects of eltrombopag include thromboembolic events (2%), mild increases in ALT levels (3%), and increased total bilirubin levels (4%).

This concludes Idiopathic Thrombocytopenic
Purpura (ITP): Fast Focus Study Guide

Search Amazon Kindle books to find other study
guides written by

JT Thomas, MD

Internal Medicine Study Guide

Hematology Study Guide

Medical Oncology Study Guide

Cardiology Study Guide

Multiple Myeloma Study Guide

Differential Diagnosis Study Guide

Rheumatology Study Guide

Cancer Study Guide

www.ingramcontent.com/pod-product-compliance
Lightning Source LLC
Chambersburg PA
CBHW070929180526
45168CB00003B/1006